Cancer and people with learning disabilities

The evidence from published studies and experiences from cancer services

James Hogg, John Northfield and John Turnbull

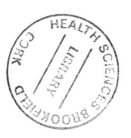

Acknowledgements

The production of this publication was supported by a grant from the Department of Health.

British Library Cataloguing in Publication Data
A CIP record for this report is available from the Public Library

ISBN 1 902519 73 6

BILD Publications is the publishing office of the
British Institute of Learning Disabilities
Wolverhampton Road
Kidderminster
Worcestershire
United Kingdom
DY10 3PP
Telephone: 01562 850251
Fax: 01562 851972
e-mail: bild@bild.demon.co.uk
Website: www.bild.org.uk

Please contact BILD for a free publications catalogue listing BILD books, reports and training materials.

BILD Publications are distributed worldwide by
Plymbridge Distributors Limited
Plymbridge House
Estover Road
Plymouth
United Kingdom
PL6 7PZ
Telephone: 01752 202301
Fax: 01752 202333

Preface

This review was commissioned by the Department of Health to provide background information for "Valuing People: a New Strategy for Learning Disability for the 21st Century"[1] – the Government's strategy for people with learning disability in England. One of the central aims of this strategy is to enable people with learning disabilities to derive full benefit from mainstream services of the National Health Service, including primary and secondary healthcare. The Government has committed additional resources to the NHS and National Service Frameworks and these are now in place for mental health, for coronary heart disease, for children, and for older people. The National Cancer Plan, which is now being implemented, makes specific reference to the needs of people with learning disabilities. But we are remarkably ignorant about cancer in people with learning disabilities and if we are to provide a health service worthy of the 21st Century then we need to know much more about the potential genetic, environmental and personal risks to which people with learning disabilities may be exposed. We need to ensure that health education programmes are accessible to people who may have problems in understanding the written word. Because people with learning disabilities may not be able to report their symptoms we also need to know how to improve rates of early diagnosis through regular surveillance and health checks. We need to achieve a better understanding of how to ensure that people with learning disabilities co-operate with the complex treatment regimes now deployed to treat cancer. Finally we need to understand more about how to deliver high quality palliative care.

In commissioning this review we did not expect to find answers to all the queries. We were looking firstly for a review of the scientific literature that would provide a platform for the future. James Hogg has provided us with just what was needed – a comprehensive, yet succinct overview of the scientific literature. Secondly, we wanted to learn from the experience of people with learning disabilities, their carers and those who provide cancer services about the impediments that lie in the way of providing good quality provision. John Turnbull and John Northfield have assembled the views of people who have had experience in planning and commissioning cancer services as well as those who have been providers.

I hope that this book will stimulate readers to develop the knowledge, diagnostic competencies and skill base that will be needed if people with learning disabilities are to have access to high quality cancer diagnosis and treatment.

Oliver Russell
Chairman of Trustees
British Institute of Learning Disabilities

---

[1] Department of Health (2001) Valuing People: A New Strategy for Learning Disability for the 21st Century. London: The Stationery Office Cm 5086.

Contents:

Part 2

PART I

The Evidence from Published Studies

James Hogg

Summary: Part I

The published literature that deals with, or refers to, cancer and people with learning disabilities is reviewed. Attention is drawn to the pervasive finding that both morbidity and mortality among people with learning disabilities are most frequently related to respiratory and cardiovascular conditions, with the prevalence and incidence of cancer some way behind. Conclusive epidemiological information regarding prevalence and incidence with respect to morbidity and mortality is lacking, however.

Though changing life style arising from increased choice in community settings and greater longevity has been predicted to lead to an increase in cancer in this population, specific evidence is lacking. There is no unequivocal information on trends in the prevalence and incidence of cancer. With respect to specific causation, a persistent finding in the national and international literature is the high incidence of gastrointestinal cancer which has been linked to the high rate of *Helicobacter Pylori* in institutional populations of people with learning disabilities. The implications of this situation for community provision as institutions are closed are noted.

Specific associations between given syndromes and the occurrence of different types of cancer are noted for Down syndrome, tuberous sclerosis, Wilm's syndrome and other rare, genetic conditions. The high incidence of leukemia in people with Down syndrome receives particular attention, as does their unique tumour profile.

With respect to health promotion and surveillance the limited literature indicates that people with learning disabilities are poorly served, with significant shortcomings in screening for breast and cervical cancer in women. The literature identified important issues to do with breaking the news on cancer to people with learning disabilities and their carers, treatment strategies, and the delivery of palliative care. The last issue particularly is judged to merit fuller exploration.

Recommendations regarding the need for future research are suggested.

1 Introduction

Following *The Health of the Nation Strategy* (Department of Health 1992[1]), cancer represents one of five key health problems in the Department of Health document, *The Health of the Nation: A strategy for people with learning disabilities* (Department of Health 1995[2]). Here cancer is placed alongside coronary heart disease and stroke, HIV/AIDS and sexual health, accidents and mental illness as a principal focus of concern demanding a response based on appropriate delivery of healthcare, health promotion and health surveillance. The direct translation of priorities for the general population to people with learning disabilities has been questioned by Turner & Moss (1996[3]), who suggest that there are other priorities such as sensory impairment and dental health that meet the criteria for key area status. Certainly the general health surveys on which part of this report is based indicate that respiratory disorders are the principal cause of death – some way ahead of cancer and the other priority areas. Nevertheless, the occurrence of cancer among people with learning disabilities is a major cause of concern as it is for the general population, and merits consideration in its own right.

There are, however, two further reasons why there is increased concern regarding possible *trends* in the incidence of cancer and consequent mortality among people with learning disabilities. These relate to the changing lifestyles of many people with learning disabilities, and to the now clearly documented increase in life expectancy in this population.

For many people with learning disabilities, changing lifestyle has followed from their move from institutional provision to community living (Emerson & Hatton 1994[4]) and a far more liberalised environment. It has been suggested that with its increased emphasis of choice and individual freedom, this will expose individuals to greater health risks including carcinogenic agents, e.g. through smoking. For those who have always lived in the community, family attitudes to choice may be becoming more liberal, and certainly a move from the family home to a managed community setting may have such a consequence. Again, exposure to health risks may ensue.

Second, longevity of people with learning disabilities has increased appreciably in recent decades (For a summary of some key international references see Hogg et al 2000[5]). Even where life expectancy is less than average, as in the case of Down syndrome, there has still been a highly significant increase. This very positive development raises questions regarding the relation between age and a variety of

1. Department of Health (1992) *The Health of the Nation Strategy*. London: HMSO.
2. Department of Health (1995) *The Health of the Nation: A strategy for people with learning disabilities*. London: HMSO.
3. Turner, S. & Moss, S. (1996) The health needs of adults with learning disabilities and the *Health of the Nation* Strategy. *Journal of Intellectual Disability Research*, 40, 438–450.
4. Emerson, E. & Hatton, C. (1994) *Moving Out: Relocation from hospital to community*. London: HMSO.
5. Hogg, J., Lucchino, R., Wang, K. & Janicki, M. (2000) Healthy Ageing – Adults with Intellectual Disabilities: Ageing and social policy. Geneva: World Health Organization.

diseases, most apparently, dementia (Janicki & Dalton 1999[6]). In the general population age has been described as the most important descriptive determinant of cancer (Groenwald et al 1992[7]). While certain common cancers show highly significant increases with age (Cooper 1992[8]) some, such as Wilm's tumour and lymphocytic leukemia are cancers of childhood. With respect to the ten commonest cancers, Lamont et al (1990[9]) indicate that at any age the morbidity of a particular stage or extent of cancer is likely to be similar. However, age related differences in incidence do exist. Prostate cancer in men may be viewed as a disease of older age (Groenwald et al 1992[7]). For women, the incidence of breast cancer increases with age, as does that of colorectal, stomach and skin cancer in the whole population.

As life expectancy has, and does, increase, it may be that people with learning disabilities will as a group reflect similar trends. Where there is increased risk of a type of cancer, they too may be subject to this age-related risk. However, this cannot be assumed as significant differences in their life style, life experiences, and medical treatment over the years may result in a different picture. For example, (Evenhuis et al 2000[10]) draw attention to the interaction between high frequency chronic conditions, such as untreated childhood-onset oesophagitis, and adult disease, in this example, oesophageal cancer. From this perspective then, there will be no substitute for epidemiologically sound studies of cancer in this population as it ages. To anticipate with respect to the present review, we have found little that bears on this question.

Superimposed on the over-arching issues of changing lifestyle and ageing is the heterogeneity of the people with learning disabilities. This is not, of course, to suggest that the general population is homogeneous with respect to life style or genetic makeup. However, the population of people with learning disabilities is known to include people with highly specific genetic endowments and a certain amount *is* known about their vulnerability or otherwise to cancer. Below we deal with cancer and Down syndrome and with tuberous sclerosis, as well as a few less well known conditions that have received some attention in the literature.

The surveys we review below suggest a number of questions with respect to cancer in this population which are deceptively simple:

- What is the incidence of cancer among people with learning disabilities, and what is the relative contribution of cancer to mortality?

6. Janicki, M.P. & Dalton, A.J. (eds.) (1999) *Dementia, Aging and Intellectual Disabilities: A handbook.* Philadelphia: Brunner-Mazel.
7. Groenwald, S.L., Frogge, M.H., Goodman, M. & Yarbro, C.H. (1992) *The Cancer Problem: Part 1 from Cancer Nursing Principles and Practice. Second edition.* Boston: Jones & Bartlett.
8. Cooper, G.M. (1992) *Elements of Human Cancer.* Boston: Jones & Bartlett.
9. Lamont, D.W., Gillis, C.R. & Caird, F.I. (1990) Epidemiology of cancer in the elderly. In F.I. Caird & T.B. Brewin (eds.) *Cancer in the Elderly.* London: Wright, pp. 9–15.
10. Evenhuis, H., Henderson, C.M., Beange, H., Lennox, N. & Chicoine, B. (2000) *Healthy Ageing in People with Intellectual Disability: Physical health issues.* Geneva: World Health Organisation.

- Does the incidence of cancer differ among people with learning disabilities from members of the non-learning disabled population?

- Is the tumour profile of people with learning disabilities different from that of the general population?

- Is the incidence of cancer changing, and if so, how does this reflect changes in life style of people with learning disabilities?

- Is the incidence of cancer related to where people live?

- Are there differences in incidence related to degree of learning disability?

- Is aetiology related to incidence and types of cancer?

- What is known about women with learning disabilities and cancer?

- Is healthcare surveillance with particular reference to cancer adequate for people with learning disabilities?

- What information do we have on the effectiveness of healthcare promotion on cancer inducing behaviour and morbidity and mortality?

- What further research is required?

In general, work in this field has concerned itself with cancer as a cause of death, rather than with the incidence of the disease among the living.

It is important at the outset of this paper to signal clearly that some of these questions have not been adequately addressed in the published literature. The methodology employed to consider cancer (and other diseases) is highly variable with respect to the indices used, the settings in which people live are diverse, and, from an epidemiological standpoint, the designs employed vary markedly. To these considerations may be added the observations that the life histories of cohorts in the available studies vary markedly with respect to the country in which they live and where they have spent their lives. The most obvious consequence of this state of affairs is that given the limited number of studies, comparing like with like to establish a concensus is extremely difficult. All of these points will be apparent in the following review of relevant studies.

2 Literature Search Strategy

The review is based on published studies or reports that have appeared in journals over the past 25 years. No attempt was made to identify or search the gray literature, ie unpublished reports, that may have referred to cancer, though background documents from government departments *were* reviewed and cited where relevant. Principal databases searched were: CINAHL; Medline; PsycLit; CANCERLIT; British Nursing Index; RCN Journals Data Base. A small number of pre-prints of papers accepted for publication was received.

Though these searches focused on cancer (and associated terms) in relation to "learning disability" (and associated terms "intellectual disability"; "mental retardation", "mental handicap"), specific searches were made with regard to emerging topics, e.g. "Down syndrome" and "cancer" and "leukemia", "Wilm's tumour".

It became apparent at an early stage that references to cancer could occur in papers concerned with mortality in people with learning disabilities, and, to a lesser extent, prevalence studies of morbidity, and that these were not being identified through the computerised searches. This necessitated hand searches of a large volume of papers on mortality to identify references to "cancer" and related terms. Similarly, papers addressing health issues for people with Down syndrome were scanned for references to "cancer" and "leukemia". In the papers on mortality and learning disabilities, however, cancer rarely figured as a principal issue and was not referred to in abstracts. For example, Hayden (1998[11]) summarises in tabular form eleven US studies of mortality. In only two of these does "cancer" appear as a cause of death. (Both papers had been identified prior to consulting Hayden and are reviewed below.)

Neither the extent of the publications nor the quality of much of the data and its analysis reported merited undertaking a conventional systematic review (Chalmers & Altman 1995[12]).

3 Incidence and prevalence in the overall population of people with learning disabilities

3.1 Studies in institutions

The majority of available studies of cancer in the learning disability population have been undertaken in institutional settings or with people with an extensive history of living in a long stay hospital or some form of large congregate care setting. The longest period of study has been with respect to the mortality of residents of the Stoke Park group of hospital (UK) over a 65 year period, from 1930–1995, the results being based on information on cause of death as given in hospital records. Jancar & Jancar (1977[13]) reported a rising incidence of death from cancer from 1936–1975, though this was judged to be lower than for the general population. This finding was

---

11. Hayden, M.F. (1998) Mortality among people with mental retardation living in the United States: Research review and policy application. *Mental Retardation*, 36, 345–359.
12. Chalmers, I. & Altman, D.G. (1995) *Systematic Reviews*. London: BMJ.
13. Jancar, M.P. & Jancar, J. (1977) Cancer and mental retardation (a forty year review). *Bristol Medico-Chirurgical Journal*, 92, 3–7.

confirmed by Carter & Jancar (1983[14]) covering a fifty year period, 1930–1980. A subsequent study (Jancar 1990[15]) confirmed the rising trend during the decade 1976–1985. During this period 17.5% of deaths (53/302) resulted from cancer. None of the 24 Down syndrome residents who had died did so because of cancer. Jancar (1990[15]) comments that there was an increase in cancer of all types (i.e. gastrointestinal, breast, gall bladder, liver, uterus, bladder, bronchus, kidney, thymus and Hodgkin disease), though data to support this report are not presented. These findings were extended by Cooke (1997[16]), confirming lower incidence than in the general population, but also a drop in incidence over the last ten years of the study. Cooke reports an overall incidence of death from cancer from 1986–1995 of 13.6%, as compared to 26% reported in the general population in the *Registrar General's Annual Statistics 1986–1992*. One case of cancer was found in a person with Down syndrome, the first for 60 years. Also in a predominantly institutional sample, but employing autopsy findings, Cole et al (1994[17]) reported on causes of death over an eight-year period (1983–1991). Of the 60 cases, four deaths were reported as resulting from cancer, one of which was in a person with Down syndrome. A further institution-based study confirmed this picture with the principal causes of mortality over a 10-year period (1981–1990) being shown to be non-tubercular respiratory tract infection and cardiovascular disease (Puri et al. 1995[18]). Cancer accounted for 15.4% of deaths. Though the authors comment that the proportion of residents dying from cancer had increased "*with time*" (p.445), no evidence is cited to support this claim nor is any direct reference made to other studies as the basis on which this claim is made.

Several studies have been conducted in the United States on mortality in institutional settings and following relocation to the community. O'Brien et al (1991[19]) employed a cross-sectional design from 1974–1985 using ICD categories. Given the low turn over of residents, this had a strong longitudinal component. O'Brien et al comment on the dangers of using crude mortality rates for the entire population and consider mortality by both age and degree of learning disability. Of 165 deaths during this period, three were listed as having cancer as the *primary* cause of death, though 19 individuals were reported as having had cancer. Over the period, 1.8% of deaths resulted from cancer, appreciably behind respiratory causes (41.8%) and heart disease (37.0%). Both these causes were strongly linked to degree of disability, with heart disease predominating in people with mild-severe learning disabilities and respiratory disease in those with profound learning disabilities. No such association was found significantly for any other condition, including cancer, though this was reported as being more frequent among residents with mild-severe learning disabilities than those

14. Carter, G. & Jancar, J. (1983) Mortality in the mentally handicapped: A fifty year survey at the Stoke Park Group of Hospitals (1930–1980). *Journal of Mental Deficiency Research*, **27**, 143–156.
15. Jancar, J. (1990) Cancer and mental handicap: A further study (1976–1985). *British Journal of Psychiatry*, **156**, 531–533.
16. Cooke, L.B. (1997) Cancer and learning disability. *Journal of Intellectual Disability Research*, **41**, 312–316.
17. Cole, G., Neal, J.W., Fraser, W.I. & Cowie, V.A. (1994) Autopsy findings in patients with mental handicap. *Journal of Intellectual Disability Research*, **38**, 9–26.
18. Puri, B.K., Lekh, S.K., Langa, A., Zaman, R. & Singh, I. (1995) Mortality in a hospitalised mentally handicapped population: a 10-year survey. *Journal of Intellectual Disability Research*, **39**, 442–446.

with profound learning disabilities. O'Brien et al's result is consistent with Cooke (1997[16]) in reporting a decrease in incidence of cancer within the institution over the study period. It is hypothesised that deinstitutionalisation has led to more able individuals being moved to community settings leaving a less impaired, but also less cancer-vulnerable population behind, i.e. individuals with profound learning disabilities. The corollary of this explanation is that those who are relatively more vulnerable to cancer will now be living in the community.

A further European study parallels those of Cooke and of O'Brien et al. Raitasuo et al (1997[20]) analysed mortality data from residents of a Finnish institution (settlement) between 1972–1993 using ICD–9 definitions. They report results with respect to both the immediate cause of death, i.e. the disease, defect or disability, according to the signs of which the patient had died, and the primary cause of death, i.e. the disorder or disability which has initiated the set of diseases leading to the immediate cause of death. Again, respiratory causes predominated as the most frequent immediate cause of death, followed by vascular disease. In only 4% of deaths was a tumour the immediate cause of death. In 6% of deaths a tumour was the primary cause. While death as a result of cancer was similar to that in the general Finnish population in 0–14 year olds, it was half that expected for the general adult population. As in Cooke's and in O'Brien et al's studies, Raitasuo et al invoke deinstitutionalisation with its consequence for a more disabled population remaining in the institution as an explanation for the lower incidence of cancer.

3.2 Community and mixed population studies

The consequences of the transition from institution to community, however, remain a pertinent question. This has been explored in a series of controversial studies undertaken in California that have reported that, in this US context, mortality is significantly higher in community than institutional settings (Strauss et al 1998a[21]; Strauss et al. 1998b[22]; Shavelle & Strauss 1999[23]). While these findings have been challenged (O'Brien & Zaharia [24]) it is important to note that the authors emphasise that from their perspective their findings indicate the need for continuous, consistent and competent medical care and supervision in the community, a contribution to, not a critique of, care in the community. With respect to the impact of deinstitution-alisation on cancer mortality, however, they are not illuminating. Among the 45 people (out of 1,878) who died between 4/1993–2/1996, Strauss et al. (1998b[22]) found

19. O'Brien, K.F., Tate, K. & Zaharia, E.S. (1991) Mortality in a large Southeastern facility for persons with mental retardation. *American Journal on Mental Deficiency*, **95**, 397–403.

20. Raitasuo, J., Mölsä, S., Raitasuo, S. & Mattila, K. (1997) Deaths among the intellectually disabled. *Journal of Applied Intellectual Disability Research*, **10**, 280–288.

21. Strauss, D., Shavelle, R., Baumeister, A. & Anderson, T.W. (1998a) Mortality in persons with developmental disabilities after transfer into community care. *American Journal on Mental Retardation*, **102**, 569–581.

22. Strauss, D., Anderson, T.W., Shavelle, R.M., Sheridan, F. & Trenkle, S. (1998b) Causes of death of persons with developmental disability: Comparison of institutional and community residents. *Mental Retardation*, **36**, 360–371.

23. Shavelle, R. & Strauss, D. (1999) Mortality of persons with developmental disabilities after transfer to the community. *American Journal on Mental Retardation*, **104**, 143–147.

24. O'Brien, K.F. & Zaharia, E.S. (1998) Recent mortality patterns in California. *Mental Retardation*, **36**, 372–379.

no deaths from cancer in their community sample. During 1996, however, of 36 deaths (among 1,812 people), there were four deaths from cancer (Shavelle & Strauss 1999[23]). In the former report respiratory and then cardiovascular disease remain the primary causes of mortality.

A further longitudinal study has been reported from the Netherlands, albeit on a mixed institutional and community population (Schrojenstein Lantman-de Valk et al 1997[25]; also published as Chapter 2 of Schrojenstein Lantman-de Valk 1998[26]). Here physicians used diagnostic categories based on a questionnaire devised specifically for the study. The prevalence of health problems as well as three-year incidence rates (1990–1993) are reported. No cases of cancer are reported in either community or institutional samples, a total of 1,602. Significantly, in focusing on the need for screening, no reference is made to screening for cancer in women or men. In further work by this group (Schrojenstein Lantman-de Valk et al 1996[27]; also published as Chapter 5 of Schrojenstein Lantman-de Valk 1998[28]) references is made to the association between Down syndrome and leukemia, see 4.1 on page 22).

Given the association between increasing age and incidence of cancers in the general population, it is relevant to comment on two further studies from the Netherlands (Maaskant & Haveman 1989[29]; Haveman et al 1989[30]); also published respectively as chapters 3 and 4 of Maaskant 1993[31]). Although cancer is mentioned in Maaskant & Haveman 1989[29] as one of the diseases included in the study, no further reference is made to the condition and it is not included in the 18 disorders for which age-specific prevalences are provided.

A further community study undertaken in the UK by Cooper (1998)[32] compared physical health in a young group with learning disabilities (mean 39.2 years) and an older group (mean 73.2 years). Data were collected through interview and physical examination. No diagnoses of cancer were made in either group. It is possible that this reflected the non-invasive nature of the physical examination which might have failed to detect cancer, and/or the sample size. It is clear, however, that even if non-detection of cancer is a consequence of the study design, cancer had not previously

25. Schrojenstein Lantman-de Valk, H.M.J. van, Akker, M. van den, Maaskant, M.A., Haveman, M.J., Urlings, H.F.J., Kessels, A.G.H. & Crebolder, H.F.J.M. (1997) Prevalence and incidence of health problems in people with intellectual disability. *Journal of Mental Deficiency Research*, **41**, 42–51.

26. Schrojenstein Lantman-de Valk , H.M.J. van. (1998) *Health Problems in People with Intellectual Disability: Aspects of morbidity in residential settings and in primary health care.* Maastricht: University of Maastricht.

27. Schrojenstein Lantman-de Valk, H.M.J, van. (1996) Comorbidity in people with Down's syndrome: A criteria-based analysis. *Journal of Intellectual Disability Research*, **40**, 385–399.

28. Schrojenstein Lantman-de Valk , H.M.J. van. (1998) *Health Problems in People with Intellectual Disability: Aspects of morbidity in residential settings and in primary health care.* Maastricht: University of Maastricht.

29. Maaskant, M.A. & Haveman, M.J. (1989) Elderly residents in group homes for people with mental handicap in the Netherlands. *Australian and New Zealand Journal of Developmental Disabilities*, **15**, 219–230.

30. Haveman, M.J., Maaskant, M.A. & Sturmans, F. (1989) Older Dutch residents if institutions, with and without Down syndrome. *Australian and New Zealand Journal of Developmental Disabilities*, **15**, 241–255.

31. Maaskant, M.A. (1993) *Mental Handicap and Ageing.* Dwingeloo: Kavanah.

32. Cooper, S-A. (1998) Clinical study of the effects of age on physical health of adults with mental retardation. *American Journal on Mental Retardation*, **102**, 582–589.

been diagnosed in any of the 207 people examined. Again, respiratory and cardio-vascular diseases are cited among a range of other relatively high frequency conditions. Similar findings were reported in an earlier, comparable Australian study in which 71% of individuals were living in the community (Beange et al 1995[33]). No cases of cancer were reported, with cardiovascular problems looming large, though unusually, respiratory illness was not as salient as in other studies.

Kastner et al (1993[34]), followed up 14 deaths in a US community population of 1,300 people with learning disabilities between 1984–1988. Cause of death was classified as avoidable, potentially avoidable, or unavoidable. Two deaths as a result of cancer were reported, cancer of the cervix/uterus and Hodgkin disease. Service issues related to the cause of death were also identified, with the former judged "avoidable", the latter "unavoidable". We return to this study in a consideration of screening in Part 2, Section 4.

3.3 Learning disability and cancer type

Several of the studies reviewed with respect to incidence list the specific cancers reported as cause of death. None draw any general conclusions with respect to possible tumour profiles for the general population of people with learning disabilities and would add nothing of note to the list of the conditions mentioned above. Some authors do point towards differences. Cooke (1997, p.315) suggests that carcinoma of the bronchus, prostate gland and breast appear less frequently than in the general population. In addition, no prostate cancer was identified in residents of the hospital in 60 years.

However, special reference must be made to a persistent finding regarding gastro-intestinal cancer in this population. Increased incidence of gastro-intestinal cancer has been reported with some consistency in institutional studies. Jancar & Jancar (1977[13]) note 58% of cancer deaths resulted from this cause compared with 25% in the general population, a figure confirmed in the Jancar (1990[15]) study, and remarkably close to Cooke (1997[16]) who noted 55%. Böhmer et al (1997[35]), also studying morbidity on an institutional population, confirmed the British findings. Their standardised morbidity ratio was 2.9 reflecting the occurrence of 20 cases for the stated person years among people with learning disabilities against an expected seven cases in the general population.

Comparable information from community populations is simply lacking. Cooke (1997[16]) discusses the possible reasons for these findings, drawing attention to the association between low serum cholesterol and cancer of the colon (Jancar et al

33. Beange, H., McElduff, A. & Baker, W. (1995) Medical disorders of adults with mental retardation: A population study. *American Journal on Mental Retardation*, **99**, 595–604.

34. Kastner, T., Nathanson, R. & Friedman, D. (1993) Mortality among individuals with mental retardation living in the community. *American Journal on Mental Retardation*, **98**, 285–292.

35. Böhmer, C.J.M., Klinkenberg-Knol, E.C., Niezen-de Boer, R.C. & Meuwissen, G.M. (1997) The age-related incidence of oesophageal carcinoma in intellectual disabled individuals in institutions in the Netherlands. *European Journal of Gastroenterology & Hepatology*, **9**, 589–592.

1984[36]), as well as dietary, drug, genetic, biomedical and biophysical factors that need to be taken into account (Cooke 1997, p.312[16]). She also notes possible predisposing disease factors as there is considerable evidence of gastro-oesophageal and chronic constipation in this group, as well as the ever-present possibility that symptoms may be overlooked until treatment is impossible. Böhmer et al (1997[35]) urge the early detection and treatment of gastro-oesophageal reflux disease and the importance of preventing Barrett's dysplasia and cancer.

Duff et al (2001[37]) have examined the proposed relation between high levels of *Helicobacter Pylori (H Pylori)* infections in people with learning disabilities in institutions and the occurrence of death from stomach cancer and perforated ulcers. They draw attention to the high rate of the bacillus *H Pylori* among people with learning disabilities (92% as reported in Scheepers et al (2000[38]) and the widely reported link to stomach cancer, gastric ulcer and lymphoma, that has led to the bacillus' classification as a class 1 carcinogen. Though unable to prove that the deaths from stomach cancer and perforated ulcers in the Stoke Park Hospital Group residents' data (which they reanalyse) are the result of *H Pylori*, they suggest that the linkage is compelling.

Several important implications emerge from this study. First, they draw attention to environmental conditions associated with the transmission of *H Pylori*. Seropositivity is directly correlated with the number of people sharing bedroom space (Mendall et al[39]). Increased drooling and sharing of utensils are hypothesised to be important means of cross-infection. The issue of vulnerability of staff and family members to infection is also raised.

With respect to the eradication of *H Pylori* among people with learning disabilities, Duff et al (2001[37]) note the reasons for gastroenterologists' reluctance to consider population based screening programmes, and the recommendation that screening should only be undertaken when patients present themselves with complaints of gastritis or related symptoms. The authors note that such a protocol specifically excludes people with learning disabilities who may be unable to report their symptoms. Instead, infection may be manifest in essentially non-verbal ways such as sleep disorder, mental health problems or challenging behaviour. They note that with the closure of large institutions the infection is no longer contained, and that the incidence of infection in community settings may be increasing. They comment that the lack of annual health checks and good quality health surveillance in the community may further worsen the prognosis for people with learning disabilities.

36. Jancar, J., Eastham, R.D. & Carter, G. (1984) Hypocholesterolaemia in cancer and other causes of death in the mentally handicapped. *British Journal of Psychiatry*, **145** 59–61.
37. Duff, M., Scheepers, M., Cooper, M., Hoghton, M. & Baddeley, P. (2001) Helicobacter Pylori: Has the killer escaped from the institutions? A possible cause of increased stomach *Journal of Intellectual Disability Research*, **45**, 219–225.
38. Scheepers, M., Duff, M., Baddeley, P., Cooper, M., Hoghton, M. & Harrison (2000) *Helicobacter pylori* and the learning disabled. *British Journal of General Practice*, **50**, 813–814.
39. Mendall, M.A., Goggin, P.M., Molineaux, N., Levy, J., Toosy, T., Strachan, D. & Northfield, T.C. (1992) Childhood living conditions and *H Pylori* seropositvity in adult life. *Lancet*, **339**, 896–897.

3.4 Mean length survival from diagnosis and age of death from cancer

Information on survival rates in people with learning disabilities and cancer is generally lacking, perhaps in part a direct result of the frequent concern with mortality. Raitsuo et al (1997[20]) reported the period from diagnosis to death in their study as 1.5 years. Age at death from cancer is highly variable, with the Stoke Park studies reporting: 56.5 years (Jancar 1990[15]) and Cooke (1997[16]) 62.0 (male) & 69.9 (female). Raitsuo et al (1997[20]) report 33 years (range 5–71 years). Shavelle & Strauss (1999[23]) report an age range of 22–74 in the four cancer deaths, mean 46.25 years. Clearly these figures will be affected by the overall age range in the study cohort and cancer types, and it is probably not possible to make a firm comment on either until a suitably stratified and diagnosed population is subject to study.

3.5 Environmental factors

Greater freedom in community settings promoted by professionals who emphasise individual choice and preference has been hypothesised as increasing risk to the health of people with learning disabilities. Turner & Moss (1996[3]) draw attention specifically to obesity, resulting from excessive eating and drinking, and the effects of tobacco use. They note the association between obesity and increased mortality from cancer of the colon, rectum and prostate in men, and the gall bladder, breast, cervix, ovary and endometrium in women. Similarly, the effects of smoking in inducing cancer are anticipated to be similar among people with learning disabilities as in the general population. O'Brien et al (1991[19]) reported the expected relation between tobacco use and cancer as a cause of death. However, no lung cancer was noted, with oesophageal and digestive tract cancers most frequent. Whether there will be an increase in the coming years in smoking among people with learning disabilities remains to be seen.

With respect to such environmental causes, it must be anticipated that this will be most likely to occur in more able people with learning disabilities, leading to an association between ability, cause of death and morbidity.

However, an environmentally transmitted cause such a *H Pylori*, discussed in detail above in Section 3.3, is unlikely to be as selective and will affect not only people with the full range of learning disabilities, but also staff and family members. Here prevention is possible through improved hygiene practices and screening to eliminate the bacillus.

Turner & Moss (1996[3]) outline service responses to offering some form of healthy lifestyle intervention or healthcare promotion, a literature in which there is now an increasing amount of information of relevance to the prevention of some forms of cancer.

3.6 Conclusions

Despite Cooke's claim that the Stoke Park Hospital studies enable us to draw some conclusions regarding incidence of cancer and trends in this population, there are significant difficulties in doing so. First, the data provided reflect the relative contribution of cancer as a cause of death. Thus, as Jancar (1990[15]) acknowledges, mortality has decreased over the 60-year study period as result of improved treatment of a number of conditions, including the elimination of tuberculosis. Inevitably then, the relative contribution to causes of mortality of cancer will increase, as found. It is interesting to note that during the period of Cooke's (1997[16]) study the average age of death in the hospitals has *decreased*, presumably as a result of more able people being discharged to the community, but also because a ceiling may have been reached over this period with respect to treatment of diseases leading to death. Second, the learning disabilities hospital population has never been representative of this entire population, most of whom have always lived in the community. For comparative purposes, then, their use to draw conclusions regarding the relative incidence of cancer – with respect to morbidity or mortality – will always be questionable. Similar points may be made regarding Raitusuo et al's comparable findings.

The Stoke Park Hospital studies have had a significant influence on reports of cancer in this population. Some caution, however, is called for. Two methodological points should be made which undermine any attempt to draw inferences about trends from these British studies. First, none are explicit with respect to diagnostic criteria, in contrast to most non-British studies in which the *International Classification of Diseases (ICD–9)* was employed. Second, there may be confounding biases arising from a failure to stratify incidence with respect to age bands within the population. No attempt is made to employ standardised mortality measures which would be widely regarded as essential if any meaningful comparison were to be made (Kramer 1988[40]). Similarly, the failure to take into account differing compositions of the various hospital populations with respect to learning disabilities may be a further confounding factor if this dimension has any association with cancer incidence. According to Muir et al (1994[41]) valid comparison of cancer trends requires, inter alia:

- the definition and content of the cancer site have not changed over time

- criteria for malignancy have not changed

- no changes in the probability that cancer will be diagnosed in a population or sub-group

- introduction of screening has not altered the probability of detection

- recording of cancer has remained equally efficient over time

- coding of cancer is consistent

40. Kramer, M.S. (1988) *Clinical Epidemiology and Biostatistics: A primer for clinical investigators and decision makers.* London: Springer-Verlag.
41. Muir, C.S., Fraumeni, J.F. & Doll, R. (1994) The interpretation of time trends. In R. Doll, J.F. Fraumeni & C.S. Muir (eds.) *Trends in Cancer Incidence and Mortality.* Plainview, NY: Cold Spring Harbor Laboratory Press, pp. 5–21.

It will be apparent from what follows that such rigour cannot be assumed in studies of cancer in people with learning disabilities. The sources of data are very disparate ranging from that collected through autopsy through to use of death certificates, to non-invasive physical examinations complemented by interviews. Few explicitly employ criteria derived from ICD categories. The influence of cohort differences is sometimes acknowledged but has not been controlled for in any comprehensive study. Muir et al (1994[41]) clearly spell out the implications of cohort differences for determining the age specific rate for cancer in a population. This is a function of the combined effects of the cumulative exposure to the carcinogen(s) responsible agents, genetic susceptibility and the countervailing protective factors, variations of such exposure in prevalence and intensity in the past, and the likelihood that the cancer will be detected at the time. Again, the studies we review are on people with learning disabilities living entirely in institutional or community settings, some combination of these, in different countries where apparently similar facilities may differ markedly, and were undertaken over a 70 year period. Clearly significant, but unanalysed, cohort effects will operate.

We noted in passing the different approaches to data collection in studies of cancer and learning disability. In the wider literature there has been much debate whether analysis of trends should depend upon incidence or mortality data. Ultimately, the quality of the data collected is the key factor. Poor quality diagnosis will lead to inaccurate information in the same way that inaccurate assessment of cause of death will. In effect, the application of rigorous inclusion criteria to the studies reviewed here with respect to data quality, whether incidence or mortality, would leave little to be discussed. We have therefore adopted an inclusive approach to the studies reviewed, commenting on where the methodology might have influenced the conclusions drawn.

A final more general methodological point needs to be added. Much of what has been said about the difficulty of determining *trends* is equally applicable to making comparisons with the general population with respect to both incidence and mortality. All studies identified have employed general population statistics to make these comparisons, i.e. studies have not been undertaken on a population which includes both people with and without learning disabilities. Different diagnostic methods will therefore have been employed and in some measure a question mark will hang over conclusions.

However, such conclusions *have* been drawn and may well be incorrect or at best premature. The suggestion in a recent review by Turner & Moss (1996, p.439[3]) that "...*there is evidence that such cases* [of cancer] *may also be on the increase*" has yet to be substantiated.

4 Cancer and specific aetiologies

The studies reviewed above have been undertaken on very heterogeneous samples both with respect to the aetiology of the learning disability and the environment of the individuals – both at the time of the study and historically. They do not typically reflect the increasing differentiation that is taking place in the study of learning disability with respect to an understanding of aetiology – not least from a genetic standpoint. With respect to the occurrence of cancer in people with learning disabilities it is important to consider this issue for a variety of reasons. First, as will be shown below, there are specific associations between the occurrence of particular cancers in people with certain syndromes – and indeed – their resistance to the development of certain cancers. Second, these linkages are in the context of genetic research that suggests hypotheses regarding the genesis of cancer that will have wider benefits to patients well beyond the field of learning disability.

It is only with the former issue that we can deal here. By far the most extensive literature we have been able to locate is concerned with Down syndrome, followed by tuberous sclerosis. However, other lower incidence conditions in which the occurrence of tumours *and* developmental delay characterise the syndrome have been reported and we note a small number of these. These syndromes may be viewed in the wider context of the population in which various hereditary cancer-prone syndromes are now being identified (Abrahams et al 1998[42]).

It is also worth noting for the sake of completion that for some individuals the occurrence of cancer and learning disability will have a common cause, e.g. exposure at an early stage of development to radiation (Miller 1999[43]).

4.1 Down syndrome

Increased survival among people with Down syndrome has for some time been explicitly linked to concern about unmasked tumour morbidity (Scholl et al 1982[44]). The link between Down syndrome and leukemia was reported some 70 years ago (Brewster & Cannon 1930[45]). This relation has been confirmed in numerous papers, with Powers & Register (1991[46]) suggesting a 20- to 30-fold greater risk of leukemia in people with Down syndrome over that in the general population. In the incidence studies reported in Section 3 a small number of people with Down syndrome were

---

42. Abrahams, P.J., Houweling, A., Cornelissen Steijger, P.D., Jaspers, N.G., Darroudi, F., Meijers, C.M., Mullenders, L.H., Filon, R., Arwert, F., Pinedo, H.M., Natarajan, A.P., Terleth, C., Van Zeeland, A.A. & van der Eb, A.J. (1998) Impaired DNA repair capacity in skin fibroblasts from various hereditary cancer-prone syndromes. *Mutation Research*, **407**, 189–201.
43. Miller, R.N. (1999) Discussion: Severe mental retardation and cancer among atomic bomb survivors exposed in utero. *Teratology*, **59**, 234–235.
44. Scholl, T., Stein, Z., & Hansen, H. (1982) Leukemia and other cancers, anomalies and infections as causes of death in Down's syndrome in the United States during 1976. *Developmental Medicine and Child Neurology*, **24**, 817–829.
45. Brewster, H.F. & Cannon, H.E. (1930) Acute lymphatic leukemia: Report of a case in eleventh month mongolian idiot. *New Orleans Medical & Surgical Journal*, **82**, 872–873.
46. Powers, L.W. & Register, M.K. (1991) Down syndrome and acute leukemia: Epidemiological and genetic relationships. *Laboratory Medicine*, **22**, 630–636.

likely to be reported, e.g. Raitsuo et al (1997[20]) who reported 3/30 cases. Powers & Register (1990[46]) also explore the association of Down syndrome with different types of leukemia and their relative incidence in young children with and without the syndrome. A further discussion of aspects of different tumours associated with leukemia, but also with lymphomas, gonadal tumours, tumours of the central nervous system, germ cell tumours, retinoblastomas, skin and other tumours in Down syndrome will be found in Satgé et al (1998a[47]).

These authors go on to suggest a specific tumour profile in people with Down syndrome (Satgé et al 1998a[47]). They propose that this consists of over representation of leukemias and global under representation of malignant solid tumours. Among the latter, however, lymphomas, gonadal and extragonadal germ cell tumours, and possibly retinoblastomas and pancreatic and bone tumours are in excess. Foetal and neonatal neoplasms are seen in excess at an early age. Under representation has been noted for neuroblastomas and nephroblastomas in young children and common epithelial tumours in adults. Satgé et al (1998b[48]) comment that the lack of neuroblastomas does not indicate a general decreased incidence of cancer in people with Down syndrome, but an under representation of a specific tumour. For several of the conditions noted as being in excess of the general population, their preponderance is higher in males than females.

Satgé et al (1998) provide an exhaustive listing of the specific tumours identified in people with Down syndrome in the extensive literature.

A persistent finding in the epidemiological literature on Down syndrome and cancer is the low incidence of breast cancer in women. This finding was noted some time ago by Oster et al (1972[49]), while in Hasle et al's (2000[50]) study no cases were identified in the large population studied. With respect to cancer and women with Down syndrome, they also note increased incidence of ovarian cancers, though this finding was not statistically significant.

Studies of the total populations of children invariably confirm the relative high incidence of leukemia in young children with Down syndrome (e.g. Mertens et al 1998[51]) and much of the literature focuses on early childhood. Satgé et al (1998) note that these findings are well substantiated for children and young adults with Down

47. Satgé, D., Sommelet, D., Geneix, A., Nishi, M., Malet, P. & Vekemans, M. (1998a) A tumour profile in Down syndrome. *American Journal of Medical Genetics*, **78**, 207–216.
48. Satgé, D., Sasco, A.J., Carlsen, N.L., Stiller, C.A., Rubie, H., Hero, B, de Berardi, B., de Kraker, J., Coze, C., Kogner, P., Langmark, F., Hakvoort-Cammel, F.G., Beck, D., von der Weid, N., Parkes, S., Hartmann, O., Lippens, R.J., Kamps, W.A. & Sommelet, D. (1998b) A lack of neuroblastoma in Down syndrome: A study from 11 European countries, *Cancer Research*, **58**, 4448–4452.
49. Oster, J., Mikkelsen, M. & Nielsen, A. (1975) Mortality and life-table in Down's syndrome. *Acta Paediatrica Scandanavia*, **64**, 322–326.
50. Hasle, H., Clemmensen, I.H. & Mikkelsen, M. (2000) Risks of leukaemia and solid tumours in individuals with Down's syndrome. *Lancet*, **355** (9199), 165–169.
51. Mertens, A.C., Wen, W., Davies, S.M., Steinbuch, M., Buckley, J.D., Potter, J.D. & Robison, L.L. (1998) Congenital abnormalities in children with acute leukemia: A report from the Children's Cancer Group. *Journal of Pediatrics*, **133**, 617–623.

syndrome, though there is less evidence with respect to adults. They note that the evidence is more fragmented, and that environmental influences may be of greater importance in adult life. Work by Hasle et al (2000[50]) has thrown light on the relation between age and cancer in people with Down syndrome in a recent study. Here 60 cases of cancer were found in a population of 2,814 individuals with Down syndrome. The incidence was higher than expected on the basis of national figures which estimated 49.8 cases. The incidence also decreased across the age range, though no cases were identified over the age of 29 years. As in Satgé et al's report, the incidence of different types of cancer in childhood varied considerably, with acute myeloid leukemia occurring to a greater degree than acute lymphoblastic leukemia.

It is beyond the scope of this report to review treatment issues with respect to Down syndrome – particularly young children – and leukemia. It is worth noting, however, that changing attitudes to the inclusion of children with Down syndrome in clinical trials (Lange et al 1998[52]) are yielding studies indicating positive outcomes to treatment with respect to certain leukemias (e.g. Lange et al 1998; Lie et al 1996[53]). The suggestion in both these papers and elsewhere (Bermudez Cortes 1998[54]); Craze 1999[55]) is that prognosis for these children is as good as, or in some cases better, than for children in the general population.

It is increasingly clear that a fuller understanding of the genetic consequences of the extra copy of chromosome 21 in people with Down syndrome will explicate the reason for this unique profile of tumours. Specifically, a fuller understanding of the DNA sequence of human chromosome 21 will, as Hattori et al (2000[56]) state, have profound implications for understanding of the pathogenesis of diseases and the development of new therapeutic approaches, including cancer.

4.2 Tuberous sclerosis

Tuberous sclerosis is a genetic condition that causes tuber like growths in the brain and frequently in other organs. It is not invariably associated with learning disability though this may vary from profound to mild impairment. Benign tumours occur in

52. Lange, B.J., Kobrinsky, N., Barnard, D.R., Arthur, D.C., Buckley, J.D., Howells, W.B., Gold, S., Sanders, J., Neudorf, S., Smith, F.O. & Woods, W.G. (1998) Distinctive demography, biology, and outcome for myeloid leukemia and myeldysplastic syndrome in children with Down syndrome: Children's Cancer Group Studies 2816 and 2891. *Blood*, **91**, 608–615.

53. Lie, S.O., Jonmundsson, G., Mellander, L., Siimes, M.A., Yssing, M. & Gustafsson, G. (1996) A population-based study of 272 children with acute myeloid leukaemia treated on two consecutive protocols with different intensity: best outcome in girls, infants, and children with Down's syndrome. Nordic Society of Paediatric Haematology and Oncology (NOPHO). *British Journal of Haematology*, **94**, 82–88.

54. Bermudez Cortes, M., Verdeguer Miralles, A., Jovania Casano, C., Canete Nieto, A., Fernandez, J.M., Ferris Tortajada, J. & Castel Sanchez, V. (1998) [Down's syndrome and leukemia] *Annales Españoles Pediatrica*, **48**, 593–598.

55. Craze, J.L., Harrison, G., Wheatley, K., Hann, I.M. & Chessells, J.M. (1999) Improved outcome of acute myeloid leukaemia in Down's syndrome. *Archives of Diseases of Children*, **81**, 32–37.

56. Hattori M; Fujiyama A; Taylor TD; Watanabe H; Yada T; Park HS; Toyoda A; Ishii K; Totoki Y; Choi DK; Soeda E; Ohki M; Takagi T; Sakaki Y; Taudien S; Blechschmidt K; Polley A; Menzel U; Delabar J; Kumpf K; Lehmann R; Patterson D; Reichwald K; Rump A; Schillhabel M; & Schudy,A. The DNA sequence of human chromosome 21. The chromosome 21 mapping and sequencing consortium. *Nature*, **405**: 6784, 311–319.

the brain, heart, skin and kidney and are more frequent than malignant tumours. However, malignant tumours do occur in people with tuberous sclerosis and renal tumours have been reported (Washecka & Hanna 1991[57]). Average age of onset among patients with tuberous sclerosis was 36 years, 20 years ahead of the average for the general population (Al-Saleem et al 1998[58]). These authors report on the occurrence of malignant renal tumours in children and young adults with tuberous sclerosis, also identifying malignant tumours beyond the kidney. Despite the average age for development noted above, they draw attention to the much earlier occurrence of malignant tumours in younger people with tuberous sclerosis. Though chronic renal failure in people with tuberous sclerosis is reported as being rare, treatment issues involving dialysis and renal transplantation have received attention (Schillinger & Montagnac 1996[59]).

4.3 Wilm's Tumour

Wilm's tumour is a malignant tumour of the kidney that usually affects children before five years of age and may also occur in the foetus. It is also, among other names, known as nephroblastoma. A fuller description of this tumour and its treatment appears in (Matthay 1991[60]). This author notes the increasingly positive prognosis with respect to recovery as treatments become more effective.

References to Wilm's tumour occur in the context of a number of rare syndromes and in association with conditions that may be characterised by varying degrees of learning disability. For example a small number of cases of this tumour have been reported in association with aniridia, and it is estimated that 1 in 70 cases of aniridia will have Wilm's tumour. The association of Wilm's tumour, aniridia, genitourinary abnormalities and learning disability (mental retardation for purposes of the abbreviation), have led to the characterisation of the WAGR syndrome (Pritchard-Jones et al 1994[61]). Most individuals with this association are reported to have moderate to severe learning disabilities (Jones 1988[62]). Similarly, there is occasional association of Wilm's tumour with Bechwith-Wiedemann syndrome, associated with mild to moderate learning disabilities, though development *may* not be delayed (Jones 1988[62]). People with Bloom syndrome, occasionally associated with mild learning disability, have also been reported to be disposed to Wilm's tumour (Jones 1988[62]).

57. Washecka, R. & Hanna, M. (1991) Malignant renal tumors in tuberous sclerosis. *Urology*, **37**, 340–343.

58. Al-Saleem, T., Wessner, L.L., Scheithauer, B.W., Patterson, K., Roach, E.S., Dreyer, S.J., Fujikawa, K., Bjornsson, J., Bernstein, J. & Henske, E.P. (1998) Malignant tumors of the kidney, brain, and soft tissues in children and young adults with the tuberous sclerosis complex. *Cancer*, **15**, 2208–2216.

59. Schillinger, F. & Montagnac, R. 1996) Chronic renal failure and its treatment in tuberous sclerosis. *Nephrol. Dial. Transplant*, **11**, 481–485.

60. Matthay, K.K. (1991) Other neoplasms and miscellaneous conditions. In H.W. Taeusch, Ballard, R.A. & Avery, M.E. (eds.) *Schaffer & Avery's Diseases of the Newborn: Sixth edition*. London: W.B. Saunders, 1025–1048.

61. Pritchard-Jones, K., Renshaw, J. & King-Underwood, L. (1994) The Wilm's tumour (WT1) gene is mutated in a secondary leukaemia in a WAGR patient. *Human Molecular Genetics*, **9**, 1633–1637.

62. Jones, K.L. (1988) *Smith's Recognizable Patterns of Human Malformation: Fouth Edition*. London: W.B. Saunders.

A syndrome characterised by the Dandy-Walker malformation which results in hydrocephalus, microcephaly and Wilm's tumour with specific genetic etiology has also been suggested (Kawame et al 1999[63]). The genetic basis of this cancer is well known, as are the reasons for spontaneous regression of Wilm's and retinoblastoma.

4.4 Learning disability and other associations with cancer

It is possible that as the rapidly increasing understanding of the genetic determinants of disorders and diseases and their association develops, so the link between learning disability and a variety of diseases, such as cancer, will become clearer. Ataxia-Telangiectasia, for example, is a condition involving neurodegeneration, recurrent infections as the result of radiosensitivity and genetic instability. Half of such children will be characterised by learning disability. Ten per cent will develop a malignancy in childhood or early adulthood, typically lymphoid leukemias or lymphomas. There is an increased risk of breast cancer in women who are carriers of AT gene mutations.

5 Women with learning disabilities and cancer

Greater opportunities to make personal choices and to lead a life in the community affect women with learning disabilities to the same extent as men. It has been suggested (Parrish & Marwick 1998[64]) that while this has resulted in increased autonomy and independence, they have at the same time become more vulnerable and in danger of lack of support and of isolation. Similarly, their increased longevity exposes them to age-related diseases, not least of which are the cancers.

Almost nothing is known, however, about the impact of their changing environment or increased longevity on the incidence of cancer among women with learning disabilities, either generally, or with respect to breast and cervical cancer (Walsh et al 2000[65]). However, in this last report as well as elsewhere, there is a growing emphasis on the right of women with learning disabilities to be included in screening programmes, particularly with respect to breast and cervical cancer.

5.1 Breast cancer

Adequate data on the prevalence or incidence of breast cancer in women with learning disabilities are lacking. We have noted the very low incidence of breast cancer in women with Down syndrome. Occurrence of the condition has been reported in several institutionally-based studies. Jancar & Jancar (1977[13]) reported 13 women dying of breast cancer, with Jancar (1990[15]) noting five women. Walsh et al

---

63. Kawame, H., Sugio, Y., Fuyama, Y., Hayashi, Y., Suzuki, H., Kurosawa, K. & Maekawa, K. (1999) Syndrome of microcephaly, Dandy-Walker malformation, and Wilm's tumor caused by mosaic, variegated aneuploidy with premature centromere division (PCD): Report of a new case and review of the literature. *Journal of Human Genetics*, 44, 219–224.

64. Parrish, A. & Marwick, A. (1998) Equity and access to health care for women with learning disabilities. *British Journal of Nursing*, 7, 92–96.

65. Walsh, P.N., Heller, T., Schupf, N. & Schrojenstein Lantman-de Valk , H.M.J. van. (2000) *Healthy aging – Adults with Intellectual Disabilities: Women's Health and Related Issues.* Geneva: World Health Organization.

(2000[65]) note that women who have never been pregnant, including those with learning disabilities, may be at higher risk.

Early detection of breast cancer remains the principal strategy for reducing mortality. Royal College of Nursing (1995[66]) suggests that women with learning disabilities may be dependent on their carers looking for relevant breast changes and that these carers will require education in how to undertake examinations. Direct assistance should therefore be given for them to participate in the National Health Service Breast Screening programme (See NHS Cancer Screening Programmes: Good Practice in Breast and Cervical Screening for Women with Learning Disabilities (2000), http://www.cancerscreening.nhs.uk/publications/bsp46-csp13.html). Specific initiatives to this end are now being reported by various NHS Trusts (see Cowie & Fletcher 1998[67]). These authors describe in some detail the implementation of a Trust-wide breast awareness and screening programme and its evaluation.

Davies & Duff (2000[68]) report that in a small scale study of women living in community group houses only half had received invitations for attendance for mammography, though when they had been invited, uptake was very high (90%). A third of women were reported to undertake monthly breast self-examination, a similar proportion being examined by GPs when no Well Woman clinic was available. Where such clinics were available, less than 20% of women had attended. This study notes the problem of ensuring women with significant learning disabilities become aware of the issues involved, and the crucial role of staff. Piachaud & Rohde (1999[69]) found that only two out of 20 women with Down syndrome has been screened for breast cancer in the previous three years and likewise emphasise the importance of health education.

5.2 Cervical cancer

The Health of the Nation: A Strategy for People with Learning Disabilities emphasises the importance of including people with learning disabilities in all surveillance and health promotion programmes available to the rest of the population. However, special difficulties in realising this aspiration are widely reported (Cowie & Fletcher 1998[67]; Holmes & Parrish 1996[70]). Pearson et al (1998[71]) found only one woman in four with learning disabilities in Exeter received cervical

66. Royal College of Nursing (1995) *Breast Palpation and Breast Awareness: Guidelines for Practice*. No. 35. London: RCN.

67. Cowie, M. & Fletcher, J. (1998) Breast awareness project for women with a learning disability. *British Journal of Nursing*, 7, 774–778.

68. Davies, N. & Duff, M. (2000) Breast cancer screening for older women with learning disabilities living in group homes. *Journal of Intellectual Disability Research*. (in press.)

69. Piachaud, J. & Rohde, J. (1999) Screening for breast cancer is necessary in patients with learning disability. *British Medical journal*, 316, 1979–1980.

70. Holmes, A. & Parrish, A. (1996) Health of the Nation for people with learning disabilities. *British Journal of Nursing*, 5, 1184–1188.

71. Pearson, V., Davis, C., Ruoff, C. & Dyer, J. (1998) one quarter of women with learning disabilities in Exeter have cervical screening. *British Medical Journal*, 316, 1979 (27 June).

screening. In response to this report, Hall & Ward (1999[72]) undertook an intensive screening programme by the Horizon (NHS) Trust Health Promotion in collaboration with the Women's Nationwide Cancer Control Campaign. This involved 128 eligible women in a hospital. Care was taken to involve carers and only women staff were involved. Successful screening proved possible for 45 women, 35% of the total. Of the other 65%, 40 were behaviourally or physically unsuitable to proceed, 25 were virgins or refused, 18 were non-co-operative. Of those successfully completed, 39 results were negative, five inadequate, and one showed an abnormality. These authors make the telling comment that it was not possible to predict which women had been sexually active, a significant point given the assumption that because a woman has learning disabilities, she is therefore unlikely to be sexually active. Low occurrence of cervical screening was confirmed by Stein & Allen (1999[73]). GPs surveyed with respect to reasons for not screening women with learning disabilities commented on their assumption that they were sexually inactive, physical and emotional difficulties with the examination and problems regarding giving consent. Essentially the same findings are reported by Djuretic et al (1999[74]) with only 19% of women reported to have received cervical screening. The figure is even lower in Whitmore (1999[75]), 14%. Here to promote sexual health care for women with learning disabilities a multidisciplinary team consisting of representatives of social services, health, education, voluntary services, carers' groups and people with learning disabilities has been established.

Wilkins (2000[76]) provides a valuable discussion of the effects of sexual abuse on the willingness of women with learning disabilities to tolerate cervical screening. She is piloting a home visiting screening service based on both her knowledge as a learning disability nurse, and specialist training in screening, aimed at this small but important group of women.

The report by Kastner et al (1993[34]), above, is of particular interest here and is illuminating in other respects with regard to screening. The case of avoidable death through cancer of the cervix/uterus is described as follows, and is quoted fully here for two reasons. First, it is one of the few individual reports in the literature on cancer in a person with learning disabilities. Second, it highlights some of the inherent problems in diagnosis and treatment of a person with learning disabilities, even when what appears to be a high quality service network is available: *". . . .a 62-year-old female with moderate mental retardation of unknown etiology who lived in a group home and presented with stage 4 cervical cancer. She died within 3 months of referral.*

72. Hall, P. & Ward, E. (1999) Cervical screening for women with learning disability. (Letter). *British Medical Journal*, **318**, 536–537 (20 February).

73. Stein, K. & Allen, N. (1999) Cross sectional survey of cervical cancer screeing in women with learning disabilities. *British Medical Journal*, **318**, 641.

74. Djuretic, T., Laing-Morton, T., Guy, M. & Gill, G. (1999) Concerted effort is needed to ensure these women use preventive services. *British Medical Journal*, **318**, 537.

75. Whitmore, J. (1999) Sefton has multidisciplinary group to promote sexual health care for these women. *British Medcial Journal*, **318**, 537.

76. Wilkins, J. (2000) Pioneering spirit. *Learning Disability Practice*, 3, 4–8.

Of note is the fact that although her medical record made no mention of sexual history, the patient has given birth to a child and had lacked routine gynecological care." (p. 288). More broadly, the avoidable and potentially avoidable deaths in this study, including this woman, were, *inter alia*, associated with: a lack of a medical history, inadequate healthcare screening, lack of community social supports, gaps in the integration of healthcare services with other community provision, and healthcare provider misjudgment.

Walsh et al (2000[65]) draw attention to a number of barriers to screening in addition to assumptions regarding sexual inactivity. Inadequate receptive and expressive language skills, and difficulties in ensuring co-operation, are among them. They note cultural differences with respect to sensitivities to genital contact that may further put women from ethnic minority backgrounds at risk.

With respect to the relative importance of breast and cervical cancer screening, Davies & Duff (2000[68]) note that the risk of death is 7:1. Given that nulliparity increases the risk of breast cancer and lack of sexual activity decreases the risk of cervical cancer, they suggest that it is breast screening that should be prioritised. Against this must be set, however, the very low incidence of breast cancer in a significant sub-group of people with learning disabilities, i.e. women with Down syndrome, and also the danger of unsubstantiated assumptions regarding sexual inactivity in women with learning disabilities. More basically, from an ethical standpoint the relevance of prioritisation to the availability of the two types of screening has to be questioned when viewed against provision for women in the general population.

6 Issues in breaking bad news to people with learning disabilities and their carers and treatment

Where a positive diagnosis of cancer *is* made, informing and supporting the person will be required. Tuffrey-Wijne (1997[77]) noted the need for carers – informal and informal – to learn about terminology. She also draws attention to the possibility that health care professionals may still hold negative attitudes towards learning disability, leading to further difficulties.

Read (1998[78]) has provided a detailed list of suggestions as to how communication can be made most effective in the palliative care relationship. She draws on the composite model of palliative care with multidisciplinary input and close involvement of the person's family.

While it would be expected that from a treatment standpoint a person with learning disabilities would receive appropriate medical interventions comparable to any other citizen, the special requirements of the situation when a person with significant

---

77. Tuffrey-Winje, I. (1997) Palliative care and learning disabilities. *Nursing Times*, **93:31**, 50–51.
78. Read, S. (1998) Breaking bad news to people who have a learning disability. *British Journal of Nursing*, 7, 86–91.

communicative difficulties has cancer merit consideration. Tuffrey-Wijne (1997[77]) and March (1991[79]) both emphasise the need to communicate with the person about the nature of their illness and also, where relevant, to assist her understanding of death.

Bycroft (1994[80]) describes the input of a Macmillan nurse to a woman with profound and multiple learning disabilities living in an institution. She describes advice to staff on pain and symptom control, wound care, nutrition and palliative care, as well as communication with the multidisciplinary team which should include the patient's family. Teaching sessions with all levels of staff, information packs on pain control, care of fungating malignant lesions and cancer nursing care were undertaken. The importance of communication through facial expressions, touch, eye contact and arm movement are noted. In this area in particular the value of input to nurse education with respect to communicating with people with learning disabilities, particularly those who are non-verbal, should be considered. This might have gone some way to alleviating Bycroft's early difficulties on which she reports with some honesty when she notes her initial failure to undertake a full assessment, which *"...may have been due to my apprehension and uncertainty about caring for someone with a severe mental as well as physical handicap."* (p.132). She emphasises: *"There is distinct lack of literature about palliative and terminal care needs of people with learning disabilities. It is unclear how well this group is integrated into mainstream palliative care services. It is possible that nurses with specialist skills in both fields could help to improve services. Research into palliative care needs of this client group would certainly be beneficial."* (p.51)

7 Inclusion in screening programmes and health surveillance

There is wide agreement that people with learning disabilities should be served by the primary and secondary healthcare services that are used by the wider population, though equally clear evidence that there are a variety of barriers to such access (Hogg 2000[81]). Among these are under reporting of illness arising from a failure on the part of carers to identify healthcare needs and communicative difficulties of the people themselves. Shortcomings in undergraduate and continuing medical education have also been reported.

With respect to involvement in screening programmes generally, and health surveillance initiatives it is clear that despite model and demonstration projects people with learning disabilities are poorly served. When we consider cancer specifically, there is little to add beyond the work reported in Section 5, above. With

79. March, P. (1991) How do people with a mild/moderate mental handicap conceptualise physical illness and its cause? *British Journal of Mental Subnormality,* 37, 80–91.

80. Bycroft, L. (1994) Care of a handicapped woman with metastatic breast cancer. *British Journal of Nursing,* 3, 126–128, 130–133.

81. Hogg, J. (2000) *Essential Healthcare for People with Learning Disabilities.* London & Dundee: Mencap, City Foundation & The White Top Research Unit, University of Dundee.

respect to both breast and cervical cancer screening the proportion of women with learning disabilities who participate is regarded as low, and special provision needs to be made.

We have already commented on the way in which people with learning disabilities may be disadvantaged with respect to existing protocols for screening for *H pylori* bacillus, a situation that requires urgent consideration given the link between *H pylori* and stomach cancer and ulcers.

With respect to preventative measures that might be achieved through adequate healthcare surveillance, it appears that both women and men are poorly serviced with respect to the diagnosis and treatment of cancer.

8 Healthcare promotion and cancer

There is a general awareness in the learning disability literature regarding environmental causes of cancer and the link to changing lifestyles. There are also an increasing number of healthcare promotion projects and a burgeoning popular literature of instructional material. There are, however, no studies demonstrating the impact of such initiatives or educational material on the incidence of cancer morbidity or mortality among people with learning disabilities. At present the best that can be suggested is that common sense and professional responsibility dictate that information on the causation of cancer be made widely available to people with learning disabilities and their carers, and advice and support on improving healthcare should be encouraged.

9 Concluding comments

9.1 *What is the incidence of cancer among people with learning disabilities, and what is the relative contribution of cancer to mortality?*

It is not possible to make a definitive statement regarding the incidence of cancer among people with learning disabilities. Published studies have been conducted with variable methods and are often methodologically weak. A small number of studies conducted in institutions have suggested that the incidence of cancer is lower in this population in such settings, though there are no epidemiological studies to demonstrate the cause of lowered incidence.

There is high consistency in the literature with respect to the principal causes of mortality among people with learning disabilities. Respiratory and cardiovascular disease emerge as the main causes, with cancer some way behind. This does not minimise in any way the importance of cancer or the need for treatment, but clearly indicates that other health improvement objectives also merit significant attention.

9.2 Does the incidence of cancer differ among people with learning disabilities from members of the non-learning disability population?

Studies attempting to address this question have typically been undertaken in institutional settings and as noted above, point to a lower incidence among people with learning disabilities. These findings may be influenced by the differing demographics of the learning disability population with respect to: (a) life expectancy (cancer is an age-related disease and the life expectancy of people with learning disabilities remains lower overall than that of the general population); (b) the population of people with learning disability is very heterogeneous with respect to aetiology and factors predisposing particular syndromes to cancer. In addition, epidemiologically many reports use unsound methods relative to the quality of studies undertaken in the wider population. With respect to comparative studies which are methodologically adequate and which have been undertaken in community settings, we simply do not know what the relative incidence of cancer in the population of people with learning disabilities is.

9.3 Is the tumour profile of people with learning disabilities different from that of the general population?

There are no comparative studies that would enable us to answer this question in a general sense. Should any be undertaken, it would be desirable to differentiate specific syndromes associated with cancer, e.g. Down syndrome, tuberous sclerosis and a range of low incidence genetic conditions. There is, however, a persistent finding – again deriving principally from studies undertaken in institutional settings – that gastro-intestinal cancer has a particularly high prevalence among people with learning disabilities. The involvement of the bacillus *H Pylori* in causation has been widely suggested. With respect to specific learning disability aetiologies, we know the incidence of certain cancers is higher (see 9.7, below).

9.4 Is the incidence of cancer changing, and if so, how does this reflect changes in life style of people with learning disabilities?

Suggestions that the incidence of cancer was rising, and also falling, have come from studies undertaken in institutional settings over a long period of time. These findings have to be set against a background of the changing composition of the institutional population as hospitals move towards closure, and methodologically no account has generally been taken of such change. Inferences that cancer will rise in community settings are based on two assumptions. First, increased longevity will raise the probability of cancer developing with increasing age; second, community lifestyles will expose people to greater risks as a result of increased smoking, less healthy diet, etc. While attention needs to be directed to ensuring that diseases of later life are adequately treated and healthy lifestyles developed, there is no explicit data at present to demonstrate an increasing trend in the incidence of cancer. The occurrence of cancer with respect to both morbidity and mortality is usually limited to a small number of cases, if any, in reports on those living in the community.

9.5 Is the incidence of cancer related to where people live?

There is no clear information on the relation between the incidence of cancer in people living in large institutions and small community dwellings.

9.6 Are there differences in incidence related to degree of learning disability?

Higher incidence of cancer in people with mild and moderate learning disabilities relative to those with severe and profound learning disabilities has been reported. The extent to which this finding has been influenced by the lower life expectation of people with more severe learning disabilities has not been determined. In addition, the occurrence of cancer in certain syndromes associated with profound learning disabilities would suggest that the question posed is somewhat simplistic and needs to be unpacked with respect to age and aetiology. Though not raised in the literature, it is possible that cancer in people with learning disabilities is under diagnosed relative to their older peers.

9.7 Is aetiology related to incidence and types of cancer?

It is clear that there are important linkages between aetiology and the occurrence and types of cancer. A different tumour profile has been demonstrated for people with Down syndrome, as has a very significantly increased risk of childhood leukemia. Specific cancers in this group have been found to have differing incidences from the general population, e.g. gonadal cancer in men is higher; breast cancer is lower in women. The link between benign and malignant cancers in people with tuberous sclerosis, particularly malignant cancers of the kidney, is well established. There are also several low incidence genetic conditions in which the occurrence of cancer is evident.

These findings suggest that future studies of incidence or prevalence of cancer in the population of people with learning disabilities should be designed explicitly to consider syndromal and aetiological differences among sub-groups. With respect to all these syndromes, specific medical surveillance is required.

9.8 What is known about women with learning disabilities and cancer?

Women with learning disabilities are vulnerable to cancer as are those in the general population. Again, any direct comparison with respect to prevalence and incidence is not possible in the light of the available information. As noted above, there is a strong indication that women with Down syndrome are less vulnerable to breast cancer than their non-learning disabled peers.

There is specific and general evidence that women with learning disabilities are not included as fully as is desirable in cervical and breast screening programmes.

9.9 Is healthcare surveillance with particular reference to cancer adequate for people with learning disabilities?

The evidence we have on involvement in screening programmes and health surveillance initiatives generally is limited, but suggests that both women and men with learning disabilities are poorly served. With respect to cancer specifically, this is certainly the case as limited evidence from studies of women and breast and cervical cancer screening indicates that only a minority receive these services. Where specific linkages have been suggested, as between stomach cancer and ulcers and *H Pylori*, people with learning disabilities who show a high prevalence of this bacillus may be particularly disadvantaged by existing medical protocols.

9.10 What information do we have on the effectiveness of healthcare promotion on cancer inducing behaviour and morbidity and mortality?

Despite a growing number of projects and publications on improving healthy life styles there is no information on the effectiveness of such interventions on reducing the incidence of morbidity or mortality in people with learning disabilities. Clearly a wider knowledge of the causes of cancer, such as smoking, dictate that support is given to people with learning disabilities and their carers so that they may make informed choices about how they care for themselves.

10 Future research

Even the limited references to research into the genetic basis of some cancers in people with learning disabilities will have indicated that profound progress will be made in this area in the coming years. It is significant that people with learning disabilities, such as those with Down syndrome, occupy an important place in contributing to this understanding through their own genetic make-up which predisposes them to both developing, or in some instances avoiding, certain types of cancer. The agenda for such work is well defined and on going, and here it need hardly be urged that continued research that will benefit all people, including those with learning disabilities, should be continued.

Where specific linkages to a given causation have been proposed – certainly with respect to that between *H Pylori* and stomach cancer and ulcers – research directed at elucidating the relation between cancer and the incidence of the bacillus is urgently needed in community settings. This could usefully be linked to approaches to the management of hygiene in settings in which cross-infection is to be anticipated.

With respect to research into treatment, it is crucial that people with learning disabilities remain a population of interest and concern, especially where special linkages between causation and aetiology have been demonstrated.

Other areas of research into cancer and learning disabilities are not as well served. Epidemiological studies as a body of work are limited by the variable methods used to consider cancer morbidity and mortality, limited time-scales, and an over-concentration on institutional populations. If incidence and prevalence of cancer are to be monitored and the impact of health surveillance and health promotion to be evaluated, further research is urgently needed. A comprehensive, longitudinal study of the incidence of cancer – morbidity and mortality – is required.

For obvious ethical reasons, however, health surveillance and health promotion initiatives cannot wait on an adequately defined epidemiology of cancer in people with learning disabilities. With respect to the former there needs to be an expansion in both incorporating people with learning disabilities into existing programmes, with evaluation of the success with which this is achieved and analysis of the factors that make this possible. With respect to health promotion, research and evaluation will continue to focus on behavioural change and improved knowledge, and the programme characteristics that lead to successful outcomes. Such initiatives should automatically include family and professional carers in most instances, both to ensure *their* education *and* to put them in a position to support the person for whom they are responsible.

Finally, it appears that the strides that have been made enabling people to cope with cancer, and the development of palliative care, have had only a limited impact on people with learning disabilities and their family members. There is a need to encourage a rapprochement between specialist cancer nursing and the experience of nurses, doctors and other relevant professionals in the field of learning disabilities. Research into the management of cancer in people with learning disabilities and appropriate training is much needed.

PART 2

Experiences from cancer services

John Northfield
John Turnbull

1 Introduction

The previous section of this report highlighted the key messages from the research literature on cancer and people with learning disabilities. This section goes on to report on the experiences of people with learning disabilities, their families and staff of cancer services. In this strand of the project, the interviews were free ranging and were based on the following questions:

a)   What information is available about cancer and cancer services and how accessible is it for people with learning disabilities?

b)   What makes cancer services work well for people with learning disabilities?

c)   Are there any barriers to screening, diagnosis and treatment for cancer for people with learning disabilities?

d)   To what extent do people with learning disabilities feel in control of their treatment and care if they have cancer?

The report sections that follow provide contextual information on the themes from respondents, some boxed illustrations from individual stories followed by some key points for further attention.

2 Method

This statement was carried out over a three month period, including 11 days which were allocated to interviews with respondents. Given the time constraints, the aim was to obtain as rich a data set as possible whilst giving a wide range of respondents the opportunity to contribute to the project. Therefore, a call for respondents was placed in a variety of journals and through conferences. The project steering group also suggested a number of key individuals and organisations who were invited to contribute (For a full list, see appendix *i*.).

The time restraints also meant that we were unable to recruit as many family members as we would have liked.

Each respondent was initially sent a questionnaire based on the questions described in the introduction to this section. Following this, a number of interviews were carried out, either face-to-face or over the telephone. Some respondents submitted information via e-mail. A number of key themes and consistent messages emerged which are presented below.

3 Access to information on cancer care for people with learning disabilities and their carers

Information about cancer is available for the public from a variety of sources that include local sources such as GP surgeries and hospitals and from national specialist organisations such as the Churchill Hospital Cancer Information Centre based in Oxford and Cancer Bacup.

From interviews with respondents, it was clear that the information available is presented in ways that are difficult for many people with learning disabilities to understand. For example, there was a lack of information in pictorial form or on audio or videotape. Exceptions include Cancer Bacup who provide information on audiotape and have just released a new version of their CD ROM. Although this is welcomed, this information is aimed at the general population. The Department of Health has published guidance and information on good practice relating to breast and cervical screening for women with learning disabilities. This will initially be published in paper format but there are plans to develop audio-visual and on-line material to support the guidance (available at www.cancerscreening.nhs.uk).

A lack of information makes explanation at the time of diagnosis difficult. For instance, a community learning disability nurse pointed out that, at the point of diagnosis of cancer being made for the woman whom she supported, there were no resources she could use to explain the implications of the disease. This made it difficult to fully involve the woman in making decisions about her treatment.

The positive impact of information designed for people with a learning disability is illustrated by Phoenix NHS Trust which has developed a pack on breast screening using large pictures and an easily understandable text. In addition, staff explore the meaning of this information via role play. Testicular and prostate cancer have also been addressed in this format by the Trust.

A related issue highlighted by Greenhalgh (1994), and partly confirmed by respondents in this statement, is that information is best received by people with learning disabilities in the context of trusting relationships (see section 5 below).

● **There is a clear need to develop specific materials on cancer for people with learning disabilities. In addition, there is a need to make this information available through local as well as national sources, including on-line access via the world wide web.**

4 Access to screening, detection and diagnosis

It is well documented (Department of Health 1995, 1998 and Howells 1997) that many people with learning disabilities experience difficulties in seeking and accessing health care support and many people rely on others to recognise changes in their health status. These difficulties extend to screening programmes for cancer. Studies by Pearson et al (1998) and Stein and Allen (1999) found that the uptake of cervical screening for women with learning disabilities was less than that for the general population. A key issue in the work by Stein and Allen was that women were considered to be at a lower risk because of assumptions about their sexual inactivity. Investigation into screening in Hertfordshire in 1997 (in Wilkins, 2000) found that 128 women were offered screening but only 45 underwent the procedure. A number were withdrawn from the process because they were viewed as unable to take part because of behavioural or physical reasons. Despite the growing amount of literature highlighting the problems of access faced by people with learning disabilities, these difficulties can be overcome by thinking more creatively about individual need. For example, Wilkins (2000) describes a scheme devised to offer cervical screening to women with learning disabilities in their own homes in order to overcome their anxieties.

Barriers to health care (Howells 1997, p 63)

- *Physical barriers e.g. wheelchair accessibility*

- *Administrative procedures e.g. appointment times, waiting rooms*

- *Communication difficulties e.g. an inability to describe symptoms clearly*

- *Attitudes of health professionals e.g. lack of confidence, limited experience, negative attitudes and assumptions*

- *Recognition of ill health may be difficult or delayed because:*

  a) *symptoms may not be easily identified*

  b) *family members/carers may not have the skills and knowledge to support individuals with learning disabilities to obtain health care or to maintain health-related behaviour*

  c) *'Problematic' symptoms (such as aggression) may be brought to the attention of services earlier - others that are equally significant (such as withdrawal, loss of interest) may not*

- *Reluctance to consider and provide the same range of treatment options as for the rest of the population because of:*

  a) *'diagnostic overshadowing' - the inability to see beyond the disability*

  b) *perceived difficulty in obtaining consent*

  c) *assumptions and negative predictions about how patients might react or co-operate*

A key point in detecting and diagnosing cancer (or, indeed, any other illness) is recognising the early signs that something is different. Most people have an internal 'yardstick' that they use to alert them to any change in their well being or functioning and to make decisions about seeking help and advice. As far as cancer is concerned, early detection and diagnosis can play a crucial role in successful treatment. For several respondents, the delay in detecting and diagnosing cancer was a major concern and many of them pointed to its serious consequences. Another concern was that the possibility of cancer as a diagnosis was not considered by doctors until quite late in the process of medical investigation. From the limited evidence, it is impossible to conclude that there is intentional discrimination against people with learning disabilities but this raises serious questions about accepted practice. It is beyond the remit of this project to explore current practice in the process of medical diagnosis. However, the findings from the previous section of this report, highlighting the prevalence of certain cancers amongst the population of people with learning disabilities and other risk factors, suggest that the diagnostic process should be modified to accommodate people with learning disabilities.

In one example, staff in a small home for people with learning disabilities had a sense of unease about one person but had been unable to "put their finger on why". Eventually, a diagnosis of cancer was made. However, the staff felt that the subsequent pace of intervention by medical staff, who had not previously known the person, was such that they no longer had the time to explain to the person what was happening or to help them take control of the situation. As a result, the person was admitted to a nursing home and died in a strange environment in which he knew no-one. The staff felt bewildered and many felt guilty that they had not acted in the best interests of the person.

In another example, a diagnosis of cancer was made only after an emergency admission to hospital following the onset of acute pain.

In the light of these findings it is suggested that services consider the following:

- **Staff supporting people with learning disabilities are provided with a reliable means of monitoring and recording the health status of individuals in a respectful and person-centred manner**

- **Research is undertaken to improve our understanding of how pain can be assessed and managed in people with learning disabilities who do not use speech to communicate**

- **People with learning disabilities are offered equal opportunities to participate in cancer screening programmes**

- **Appropriate levels of monitoring are introduced for people with conditions associated with an elevated risk of cancer, for example, children with Down Syndrome at risk of developing childhood leukaemia.**

5 Communicating the diagnosis, treatment options and consent

Many respondents in this statement drew attention to the difficulties faced by themselves and the person with learning disabilities in communicating the diagnosis of cancer. As mentioned in part 3 of this section of the report, staff and professionals referred to the lack of information specifically for people with learning disabilities. However, they also referred to their own fears and lack of information about cancer that might impair the clarity of any message. Learning disability nurses, in particular, expressed the need to understand more about cancer and the work of specialist organisations, such as Marie Curie Cancer Care, that would help them to support individuals to come to an understanding of their illness. Likewise, Macmillan nurses said they could help people with learning disabilities better by understanding the role of learning disability nurses.

The Palliative Care Network

There is a national network for the palliative care of people with learning disabilities that has a number of local networks affiliated to it. However, many respondents were unaware of the network and the support and guidance it could offer. In Gloucestershire, the local network is taking action to raise awareness, to become involved in education and to improve practice in the area.

Contact:
Linda McEnhill
National Palliative Care Network
Macmillan Cancer Services
Charing Cross Hospital
London
Tel: 0208 846 1629

A clear message from respondents was that telling a person about their illness is a process and not an event. Communicating this information could take time and respondents were concerned that this might further delay treatment options. Some respondents also reported feeling that "the medical machine" had taken over and other decisions were being made whilst they were still struggling with the best way of telling the person about their cancer. One of the issues raised was who is the best person to tell the individual about their diagnosis? For example, respondents said that the cancer specialist might have the knowledge about the disease pathway, treatment options and prognosis but was unlikely to have a close relationship with an individual or the necessary communication skills. Respondents said that in most cases, key workers were given the information by specialists but were left unsupported in breaking the news to the person. Some respondents reported that decisions had been made by specialist professionals not to inform the individual because they believed that the person would not be able to cope with their diagnosis of cancer. This left the support workers in the unenviable position of knowing the person had cancer but feeling unable or unsure about challenging this decision.

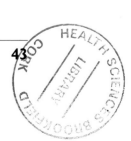

Respondents felt that the treatment offered to people with learning disabilities seemed limited to radiotherapy, chemotherapy, surgery or a combination of the three. In most cases, these treatments were presented to individuals, families and staff without question. Even though these options may have been perfectly reasonable, respondents reported that there was no consideration given to the exploration or use of complementary therapies for people with learning disabilities. Many members of the public with cancer are exploring complementary therapies, such as those offered by the Bristol Cancer Centre, that are designed to work alongside medical treatments in order to promote positive health. Respondents could not give specific reasons why complementary therapies were not considered. However, there are a number of possible explanations:

a)   support workers or families may not have information about alternatives

b)   organisations supporting people with learning disabilities may have fears about suggesting or applying complementary therapies given their duty of care

c)   the pace of medical decision making overtakes consideration of alternatives

In some cases, where it was not possible to involve the individual with learning disabilities in making decisions about treatment, respondents were concerned that the social and ethical dilemmas were not recognised or addressed. This points to the need for ongoing support for families and care staff of cancer patients with a learning disability.

A young man of 18 with learning disabilities was diagnosed with cancer and subsequently died six weeks later. The family gave their consent for chemotherapy treatment but were distressed at the impact this had on the young man's quality of life in his last six weeks. He remained in hospital during this period. After his death they were left with many uncomfortable feelings and were unsure whether they had made the right decision. They felt that their decision had not lengthened his life, nor had it improved its quality. They were supported by the primary health care team throughout but they lacked any knowledge about learning disability or how to contact the local learning disability community team. Now the primary health care team are left feeling "out of their depth" and the family are left with no counselling and a sense of bitterness about what happened.

From the accounts and opinions expressed by respondents, it was clear that clinicians do not always seek the consent of people with learning disabilities to tests and treatments. Respondents believed that the reasons for this was a desire to proceed quickly with treatment rather than a disregard of the wishes of the individual. People supporting the individual reported feeling pressured by a need for the person to receive treatment and the time it could take to explain the situation. However, other examples show that this dilemma could be resolved. A few people pointed to examples where explanations were given and consent was sought by professionals and support workers. This seemed to have taken place where organisations supporting the individual were working within a clearly expressed set of values that supported self-determination. This also seemed to extend to specialist professionals involved with the individual such as Macmillan nurses and cancer services.

Specific recommendations for improving communication are summarised below:

- Develop greater shared understanding of the respective roles of specialists in learning disability and cancer organisations

- Encourage the sharing of expertise and information in specialist areas e.g. palliative care for people with learning disabilities, pain assessment and management for people with learning disabilities

- Ensure that the same principles of communicating the diagnosis of cancer to those with the condition are applied to people with learning disabilities and that:

    a)   the news is communicated in a way that meets the communication and emotional needs of the individual

    b)   protocols are agreed locally between those supporting the individual about each other's role in communicating the diagnosis

- Ensure that the person with learning disabilities is as fully involved as possible in any decision relating to treatment and support for cancer

- Investigate the reasons why complementary therapies are not considered an option for people with learning disabilities who have cancer

- Provide information for the families and carers supporting the individual with learning disabilities

6 Planning and partnership working

A clear message coming across from the experiences of respondents was that satisfaction with services occurred when there was good partnership working between the different organisations involved in providing services and the individuals working within these organisations. There seemed to be several factors that contributed to good collaboration including:

i)   Shared knowledge of and information about different services which can contribute to the care and well being of a person with a learning disability who has cancer

ii)   A system of ongoing planning and support that placed the individual firmly at the centre of the decision making process

iii) Access to information for support workers about specialist help e.g. Macmillan nurses

iv)   The Primary Health Care Team's commitment to partnership working

v)   Good quality risk assessment and risk management plans.

One young woman lives in a residential care home and has cancer that is affecting her bones. This increases the risk that she may sustain a fracture. Within the service there is a system of person centred planning which has already recognised the need for the woman to have more information on safe and healthy lifestyles in order that she may make her own decisions. Social Services Care Managers have also been working effectively in this process.

When faced with the increased nursing need and additional risk, a risk assessment and management plan was carried out, based on the expressed wish of the young woman to remain in her home. The young woman has significant health care needs but these were discussed with the local district nursing team, Macmillan nurse and community learning disability team. As a result, the registration and inspection team was satisfied that the risk of fracture had been appropriately assessed and managed. The team meets on a regular basis to co-ordinate their input in the light of the changing needs of the young woman.

Good collaboration also seemed to stem as much from a positive organisational culture of mutual respect and knowledge of each other's roles as from specific systems or procedures. In contrast, poor experiences occurred when organisations had little knowledge of each other's roles or where responsibilities were confused. It also occurred where information was not made available to individuals or their supporters and where no-one took the lead in planning.

A woman with learning disabilities was diagnosed as having breast cancer whilst living in a residential care home. She had never had a mammogram, so the cancer was identified at a late stage. Concern was expressed within the home that staff would be unable to respond to the woman's additional nursing needs. Social Services Care Managers were not involved at this stage. A medical assessment resulted in the woman being transferred to a nursing home where she subsequently died within a matter of weeks without seeing the friends whom she had lived with.

The staff who had supported her in the residential home were left with a feeling of failure. They had not been able to care for her when they perceived her need to be greatest. It appeared that there was no attempt to plan on the basis of what was most likely to achieve the highest quality of life for the woman. There was no input from specialist palliative care staff, no care management input and the decisions seemed to

---

have been taken by 'distant' medical staff who were concerned with how easy it would be to deliver nursing support

Recommendations in relation to service planning and partnership working are:

- Local arrangements for sharing knowledge about services which can contribute to the care of people with a learning disability who have cancer.

- Promotion of a culture of person centredness in organisations so that planning and action reflects the priorities of the individual with learning disabilities

- Establishment of approaches such as Essential Lifestyle Planning to form the basis of supporting individuals with learning disabilities

- Care Management should be more connected with a person centred planning process in order to respond more effectively to changes in an individual's circumstances

7 Conclusion

This section of the report has been based on the testimony of a relatively small number of respondents. These have included direct support staff, learning disability nurses, social workers, family members, as well as some key respondents from organisations. It is a small and non-representative sample. It is not possible, therefore, to draw firm conclusions or to make very specific recommendations for action.

There are a number of clear themes that have emerged, however, where it is possible to identify issues for further investigation, research or resource development, and these have been drawn out in the emboldened bullet points at the end of each section of the report.

We did find a lack of good accessible information for people with learning disabilities about cancer, and also, where we did find some materials, staff were often not aware of their existence, and were not able to carry out systematic searches for relevant information.

Where we found examples of good practice, and cancer services working well for people with learning disabilities, this was always in the context of good quality and well established systems of person centred planning, which were able to respond to changes in individual circumstances. They were also found in the context of good quality partnership working and an effective flow of information across agency boundaries. All these aspects of effective practice can be found in the broad thrust of policy for people with a learning disability, as highlighted in the recent White Paper, Valuing People (Department of Health 2001).

We found a lot of evidence of barriers to effective screening, diagnosis and treatment, and these have been described in the body of the report. We would suggest that these barriers occur where there is a lack of knowledge, information and adequate planning systems, and it is these areas that need to be addressed if we are to bring the experience of cancer services for all people with learning disabilities to the level of the best.

The late diagnosis of cancer adversely affected patients' sense of being in control of their treatment and care. Again, where people did report that they had retained control, this was reported in the context of good quality individual planning systems.

Given the multitude of issues that have emerged from this report, there is now a clear challenge to create a more coherent and strategic response which will deliver high quality cancer services for all people with learning disabilities.

References

Department of Health (1995) "The Health of the Nation: A Strategy for People with Learning Disabilities". London, Department of Health.

Department of Health (1998) "Signposts for Success in Commissioning and Providing Services for People with Learning Disabilities". London, Department of Health.

Department of Health (2001) "Valuing People. A New Strategy for Learning Disability for the 21st Century". London, Department of Health.

Greenhalgh, L. (1994); "Well Aware: Improving Access to Health Information for People with Learning Disabilities" *NHS Executive*, Anglia & Oxford.

Howells, G. (1997); "A General Practice Perspective" in O'Hara J. and Sperlinger A. (eds.) *Adults with Learning Disabilities: a Practical Approach for Health Professionals*. Chichester. John Wiley and Sons.

Pearson, V. (1998); "Only One Quarter of Women with Learning Disabilities in Exeter have Cervical Screening", *British Medical Journal*, Vol. 318.

Phoenix NHS Trust (1995) "Getting your Breasts Screened, a Pack for Women with Learning Disabilities". Bristol, Phoenix NHS Trust.

Stein, K. & Allen, N. (1999); "Cross Sectional Survey of Cervical Cancer Screening in Women with Learning Disability", *British Medical Journal*, Vol. 318.

Wilkins, J. (2000); "Pioneering Spirit, Cervical Screening for Women with Learning Disabilities" in *Learning Disability Practice*, 3, 1, pp.4–8

Other Useful Reading

Dodd, K. & Brunker, J. (1999) "Feeling Poorly: Report of a Pilot Study Aimed to Increase the Ability of People with Learning Disabilities to understand and communicate about physical illness" in *British Journal of Learning Disabilities*, 27, 1, pp.10–15.

Matthews, D. & Hegarty, J. (1997); "The OK Health Check: A Health Assessment Checklist for People with Learning Disabilities" in *British Journal of Learning Disabilities*, 25, 4, pp.138–143.

Turner, N.J., Brown, A.R., Baxter, K.F., Turner, S. (1999); "Consent to Treatment & the Mentally Incapacitated Adult" in *Journal of Royal Society of Medicine*, 92, 6, pp.290–292.

Appendix I

DATASET

The study was carried out over a three month period including 11 days allocated to study design, delivery and interviews with respondents. The aim was to obtain a rich dataset from a wide variety of respondents. A call for respondents placed in journals and through conferences elicited a relatively small response. Clearly the issue at hand is a sensitive one for all concerned, and it proved difficult to gather more than individual personal accounts and individual experiences.

Additionally, given the time constraints it was decided not to seek information directly from people with learning disabilities, unless the opportunity arose. This is a weakness in the dataset, and should be rectified if further work were to be carried out in this area. Sufficient time for planning would need to be allocated to such a sensitive piece of work.

Because of the timescales involved, it was only possible to speak with a relatively small number of people. The table below indicates the dataset from which the report is drawn.

Individuals	
Social workers	2
Community learning disability nurses	2
General medical staff	1
Supported housing support staff	7
NHS managers	2
Family members	2

Organisations	
National Development Team	
Cancer Bacup	
Bristol Cancer Help Centre	
Macmillan Cancer Relief	
Mencap	
Norah Fry Research Centre	
Prader Willi Syndrome Association	
Down Syndrome Association	
Oncology Section, Royal Society for Medicine	
Churchill Hospital Cancer Information Centre	
Marie Curie Cancer Care Education	

Appendix II

The National Cancer Plan is a plan for investment in the NHS which will have far reaching changes across the NHS. It can be found at *www.nelh.nhs.uk* in the virtual branch library for cancer. The Department of Health will be setting national standards backed up by regular inspection by the Commission for Health Improvement. The National Institute for Clinical Excellence will ensure that the availability of cost effective drugs for cancer is not affected by where somebody lives.

The Cancer Plan also refers to Health Act Flexibilities and to the power to pool resources, or to develop care trusts, which it is hoped will prevent people with special needs falling between the two stools of health or social care organisations.

Our Healthier Nation

Cancer is a key area for the Government's White Paper, 'Our Healthier Nation'. This White Paper has a five point action plan. Below are some implications from this report for ensuring the five point action plan meets the needs of people with learning disabilities.

1 **Undertake a major review of the organisation and co-ordination of cancer research in the country**

   Professor Hogg's literature review has identified a series of strands for further research work.

2 **Appoint new cancer action team to raise standard of cancer care to that achieved by the best**

   This study clearly shows that cancer services for people with learning disabilities and their families fall far short of the best. Actions that could go some way towards improving understanding of and response to a diagnosis of cancer for people with a learning disability are summarised in the report.

3 **Extend series of guidance documents setting out best practice for individual types of cancer**

   The Department of Health has published a good practice guide for breast and cervical screening for women with learning disabilities. A recommendation of this report is that the Department of Health commissions work to develop accessible resources for people with learning disabilities about different kinds of cancer and approaches to screening, diagnosis and treatment. (Available at www.cancerscreening.nhs.uk)

4 **Commission for Health Improvement to review cancer services**

   The messages from this brief report should be fed into the Commission for Health Improvement review process, to ensure that the experience of people with learning disabilities is a part of the broader review.

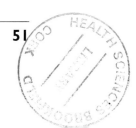

5 Undertake first ever survey of cancer patients' experiences

It will be important to ensure that there is an input from people with learning disabilities as part of the survey process referred to in 4 above. This brief study suggests that we still have a lot to learn about how cancer services respond to people who need a good deal of support, information, time and planning to ensure a high quality service response.

Appendix III

Project Steering Group

Oliver Russell
Senior Policy Advisor
Department of Health
133–155 Wellington House
Waterloo Road
London SE1

John Harris
Chief Executive
British Institute of Learning Disabilities
Wolverhampton Road
Kidderminster
Worcs DY10 3PP

Sue Carmichael
Nurse Advisor
Department of Health
133–155 Wellington House
Waterloo Road
London SE1

John Turnbull
Director of Nursing
Oxfordshire Learning Disability NHS Trust
Slade House
Horspath Driftway
Oxford OX3 7JH

Appendix IV

Messages from the Report to National Learning Disability Strategy Working Groups

This report was written to identify the issues relating to cancer and people with learning disabilities. It was written as a scoping study, to assist the Department of Health in preparing the national strategy for learning disability. The following appendix identified some of the key messages that could be addressed to the working groups developing the strategy.

The strategy has now been published as 'Valuing People' (Department of Health 2001). Some of the points in the following appendix have therefore been superseded by the publication of the white paper, but are reproduced here for the sake of completeness.

Introduction

Below are some key points from the report that can be placed against the headings of the national strategy working groups.

1 Children

There is a need to fully understand the numbers of children likely to be affected by childhood cancers, and whether there are risks associated with specific syndromes, for example the increased risk of leukemia in children with Down syndrome

(Leukaemia is from 10 to 30 times more common in Down Syndrome children than in the general population.)

Information needs to be available for families having to make treatment decisions on behalf of their child

Bereavement counselling needs to take account of the issue of negative outcome of treatment and quality of life implications during treatment

Primary care teams need to have good and timely access to information about the work of and support from community learning disability teams

2 Health

The study identified a number of barriers to diagnosis, which need work to break down. Some suggestions of areas for further work are:

Assessment of pain in people with no verbal communication;

Measures for understanding health status (eg OK Health Check);

Use of simple indicators of change in health status that might indicate warning (eg weight loss/appetite/skin changes etc.);

Work to reduce the time from seeing symptoms and making a diagnosis;

Building better relationships with primary care teams and improving the flow of information (see 'Once a Day', Lindsey M. & Russell, O. Department of Health, London, for guidance);

Creating an annotated resource packs in hard copy and on the web for (eg) screening materials;

Creating a pathway of care with links to materials to help the person, their family, supported housing carers, community team members, primary care team members, specialist cancer services staff.

Enabling the focus on the person to be maintained in the decision making process – avoid healthcare professionals making judgements about the ability of the person to deal with a diagnosis with no consultation with those who know and care about the person;

Developing and disseminating good quality and accessible resources (eg audio tapes, books without words; CD ROMs) to help support workers and families to 'break the news'.

Ensuring that current guidance on consent to treatment is available, understood and followed;

Giving support to partnership working, between primary care, specialist cancer services, residential and day support services, family members and the focus person;

Considering the implications for staff in considering alternative or complementary therapies with the focus person – what are the policy implications?

Recognising and responding to the emotional impact for staff of a diagnosis of cancer, and building in support mechanisms for them.

3 Strategy Working Group 3 – Promoting Independence

A key issue that emerged throughout the study was the perceived loss of control for the person with a learning disability when a diagnosis of cancer was made, and a feeling that the decision making process was taken over by medical practitioners who often did not know the individual, and who had had little experience of working with people with learning disabilities.

Some suggestions of areas for further work are:

Ensuring that when faced with a critical health issue like a diagnosis of cancer, often late in the progress of the disease, the person with a learning disability does not get lost in the rush to ensure that the health and medical issues are dealt with.

Ensuring that there is access to independent advocacy to help the person and their friends and family with the decision making process.

Ensuring that materials created by advocacy groups about health issues are more widely available. (Additional materials could be created working closely with advocacy groups specifically about diagnosis, treatment and care in cancer.)

4 Strategy Working Group 4 – Partnerships

Where there were examples of good practice reported by respondents to the study, they were all associated with good partnership working, including person centred planning; access to information about sources of support; Primary Care Team members committed to patient partnership; good quality risk assessment and risk management plans.

A suggestion for further work would be

Creating a clear care pathway associated with cancer care for people with learning disabilities, identifying decision points which would assist effective and timely access to information and sources of support.

5 Strategy Working Group 5 – Carers

There is considerable variability of response from different localities, and within localities at different times. This is a key theme underlying the development of the national learning disability strategy.

Some carers felt they had been put in a very difficult situation in relation to making consent decisions for their relative, where guidance about consent to treatment for adults had not been fully understood.

Access to support and counselling after the death of a relative was not always available.

Having good structures and systems were in place to involve carers in a person centred planning process was associated with the most positive responses around involvement in the decision making process relating to treatment and care options.

6 Strategy Working Group 6 – Workforce Planning Issues

Some areas for further attention might be:

Ensuring that supported housing staff have good and timely access to sources of support regarding decision making for people with a diagnosis of cancer.

Developing a clear care pathway which identifies key decision points and the kinds of help that could be available.

Recognising that staff in registered residential care settings need help to work through risk assessment and risk management procedures when people make the decision to remain at 'home' throughout the period of their illness. Staff may need additional training and support.

Developing materials to be used with people who have been diagnosed with cancer, to talk through the issues, and to help with the decision making process about treatment options etc

Helping primary care teams with appropriate access to the skills and knowledge of the community learning disability team – taking advantage of the opportunities afforded by the clinical governance agenda.

John Northfield
August 2000

about bild

The British Institute of Learning Disabilities is based in Kidderminster, Worcestershire. Supported by a national membership network of over 1200 professionals, carers, parents and enablers, BILD is committed to improving the quality of life of people with learning disabilities by advancing education, research and practice and by promoting better ways of working with and for children and adults with learning disabilities. Since its inception in 1972, BILD has become a major provider of training and publisher of books and journals on a wide range of topics relating to learning disabilities.

For more information and a catalogue of BILD publications, contact:

> **The British Institute of Learning Disabilities**
> **Wolverhampton Road**
> **Kidderminster**
> Worcestershire DY10 3PP
> Telephone: 01562 850251
> Fax: 01562 851970
> e-mail: bild@bild.demon.co.uk
> Website: www.bild.org.uk

BILD is a company limited by guarantee, No. 2804429
Registered as a charity No. 1019663